LIFE IS SWEET AGAIN

HOW I REVERSED DIABETES

Parag Shah

Non-Fiction Book Outline Template
LIFE IS SWEET AGAIN
HOW I REVERSED DIABETES
SWEETENING LIFE WITHOUT MEDICINE
PARAG SHAH

Copyright Page:

Although the author and publisher have made every effort to ensure that the information in this book was correct at press time, the author and publisher do not assume and hereby disclaim any liability to any party for any loss, damage, or disruption caused by errors or omissions, whether such errors or omissions result from negligence, accident, or any other cause.

Neither the author nor the publisher assumes any responsibility or liability, whatsoever, on behalf of the consumer or reader of this material. Any perceived slight of any individual or organisation is purely unintentional.

The resources in this book are provided for informational purposes only. It should not be used to replace the specialised training and professional judgment of a health care or mental health care professional.

Neither the author nor the publisher can be held responsible for the use of the information provided within this book. Please always consult a trained professional before making any decision regarding treatment of yourself or others.

For more information, email hitech456@gmail.com.
ISBN: (print only)

Lead Magnet:

Do you wish to reverse Diabetes organically? Then this is the book for you. Write to me at hitech456@gmail.com, and I would be more than happy to answer your queries. You would also be entitled to a free copy of my next book.

Dedication

I dedicate this book to my parents, Nalini and Subhash Laxmidas Shah, for giving my siblings and me a wholesome upbringing. Armed with the right education, ample opportunities, unconditional freedom and well-etched ideals, they paved the path for our success.

I also wish to thank all my teachers, gurus, friends and relatives for their contribution in my life.

A special thanks to Dr Pramod Tripathi, Dr Hemang Nanavati, Dr Isvar, Vasudha Chavan and all the mentors and dieticians at the Freedom from Diabetes (FFD) for this second lease of life.

This journey that took me from being non-diabetic to pre-diabetic, then diabetic and back to non-diabetic has been an eventful one. It was fraught with anxiety, anger, disagreements, fights, pressure, concern, care and much more. I understand that my family, friends and colleagues wanted the best for me, back then. However, when one is lost, one needs to find the pathway himself. So, even though I willed to come out of this challenging situation, there was no direction to my ill-concentrated efforts. Thankfully, Dr Pramod Tripathi changed that.

They say save the best for last, and I have. I am indebted to my wife, Bina and my sons, Krish and Parth for their unwavering support and faith in my unconventional methods. It wasn't easy because the fluctuating sugar levels were the anomaly. Yet, they persevered, and so did I.

And here I am with my story to tell.

Foreword

From the first time I met Parag when he joined my Turbo Sales Blueprint training, I knew he was going to be a star. He was a go-getter and had all the qualities of a leader.

One of my sessions was about book writing, and I encouraged everyone to write a book for two reasons. One, for personal branding and two, to share their learnings, experiences, and knowledge with the world. Only 10% of the students in the group could complete a book. And Parag is one of them.

In this book, Parag has shared his journey of how he reversed his Diabetes. It's no easy task. Millions of people in the world have diabetes, and they feel helpless. Starting with medicines and followed by insulin injections, many of them develop various complications like kidney failures, heart problems, and more.

Parag has proved to the world that Diabetes is a reversible disease. He has also set the path by saying if he can do it, everyone can if they know how to do so. Every diabetic person must read this book, get inspired, and get rid of this dreaded disease.

All the best, Parag. I wish you many more wins during your journey to good health.

Suresh Mansharamani

Co-Founder - Tajurba Business Network Pvt Ltd

www.SureshMansharamani.com

Table of Contents:

Introduction:

In India, we love our sweets. All celebrations must include something *'meetha'*, else is it even a celebration? However, what we miss is that in the sweetness of sugar lies the deadly sting of Diabetes.

According to the International Diabetes Federation, in 2020, over 77 million of India's population suffered from this chronic health problem. Look around, and you will find someone within your circle, living a life of fluctuating blood glucose levels.

Many of my relatives and friends have Diabetes and continue to suffer, some even to this date. They crave for certain foods and sweets, and I can't help but feel sorry for them. Despite all the efforts they put into controlling sugar, they remain powerless against this illness.

I understand their helplessness because I have been there.

At 49, my reports told me I was pre-diabetic, and that my HbA1c had crossed 6.5. Doctors advised me to start medication as a cautionary measure.

Houston, we had a problem.

No, not that I was pre-diabetic but the fact that I wasn't willing to start medication. You see, I had seen many of my friends and relatives suffer on their journey with sugar control. Their dosage kept increasing, as did their appetite for food and sugar. Their ineffective progress made me realise that popping tablets wasn't perhaps the right way to go, at least for me.

So I began looking at alternative therapies.

My journey of the next seven years from 2012 to 2019 is summarised below.

1. Soaked methi (fenugreek) seeds overnight and ate them in the morning.
2. Soaked bhindi (okra) overnight and drank the sticky water in the morning.
3. Consumed haldi (turmeric) twice, every morning and night.
4. Drank karela (bitter gourd) juice.
5. Drank dudhi (bottle gourd) juice.
6. Attempted to have no sweets but to no avail.
7. Exercised now and then, but too infrequently.

As the saga continued, so did my statistics.

In 2015 my Hb1Ac was 6.8.
In 2016, it crossed 8.
All those who loved me began insisting that I start medication immediately. Doctors warned me of dire consequences for being obstinate, yet, I held on to my beliefs. And that was for a good reason.

I had never seen anyone reduce their dosage or be free from Diabetes in my lifetime. More often than not, the patients developed other complications as well. It might not have been due to Diabetes, necessarily, but these patients had no respite. I am not against any medical system, and these are simply my observations.

I was sure that my methods would bear fruit, eventually.

Finally, in July of 2019, my wife Bina forced me to undergo one more test. It came with a pre-condition that if my Hb1Ac were more than 8, then I would start medication without further delay.

Cue the drumroll, please because my Hb1Ac was

..

..

10.3

I had no alternative but to join the fraternity of Diabetes patients forever unless I did something drastic! I had promised my wife, so I simply did what was in my best interest.

I went ahead and picked DRASTIC.

And today, I am sugar-free with my Hb1AC at 6. I have lost 16 kgs of weight (fat) and added 2 kgs in muscle. I feel more energetic, fitter and happier. I can eat sweets, and most importantly, my wife doesn't hold a grudge for not keeping my promise, back then.

How did I do it?
What were the changes?
When did the results show?

This book is an attempt to answer all these questions and more. If you or anyone you know suffers from Diabetes and are willing to bring about a change in your life, sans medicines, then walk this journey with me. I assure you, this has a sweet ending, well within the blood glucose levels.

Parag Shah

Chapter 1 : SOWING THE INTENTION

"Quantum science suggests the existence of many possible futures for each moment of our lives. Each future lies in a state of rest until it is awakened by choices made in the present".

A clear cut intention, that's what I had right from the start. I wanted a healthy life but without medicines. And I'll tell you why. I believe that the human body is a fantastic living structure with the power to heal itself. Like every efficient mechanism, you enable it with the right tools for seamless living.

I exercised for almost five days a week, with 45 minutes of brisk walk and 30 minutes of Yoga and stretching. However, neither my sugar nor my weight was under control. I was 86 kgs and 176 cm in height, giving me a BMI of 27.2. (Ideal BMI parameter was between 18-24)

Tulsi Bhai, a 60-year-old gentleman, was my garden exercise partner. He ran 10kms thrice a week and was an active marathoner. He wasn't overweight, yet he was on a strict diet and popped at least ten pills a day to control his blood sugar levels. Somehow, medication and Diabetes seemed to be in a symbiotic relationship which didn't bode well for Tulsi Bhai, at all.

One fine day, Tulsi Bhai announced he had made a shift in his exercise and diet. We acknowledged his efforts but thought nothing much of it. You see, we had succumbed to this way of life. Three months later, Tulsi Bhai made the grand announcement that his sugar levels were under control sans medicines. That's when we sat up and took notice. Was it possible?

We all put forth our debates and doubts, but Tulsi Bhai stood his ground. I was the curious one, and so I asked him the inevitable questions. He patiently answered each one as detailed as he could. I was convinced that this was a temporary solution and decided to wait it out before I made a decision.

But I didn't have to wait too long. July 2019, my Hb1AC shot up to 10.3, and as promised to my wife Bina, I had to start medication.

So, I called up Tulsi Bhai again. This time I was attentive and took his advice seriously.

In my pursuit of non-dependency on medication, I had heard of at least three methods which claimed to have reversed Diabetes for many patients. Tusli Bhai suggested one of them. I was out of options and running out of time. Ergo, I decided to go for it. There was a slim chance that this would work against the other possibility   of being on medication for life. I took the plunge with faith.

I attended the introduction seminar of the Diabetes Management process, and it made sense to my rationality. I decided to make an honest, wholehearted attempt. It was my health and well-being on the line, and I needed to be invested in it. The core of all change begins with the acceptance of 'what is' and the willingness to explore 'what if'.

I was determined to make it work this time.

I knew consistency was the key. I decided to take it one day at a time and keep on the path prescribed by the system. They say from little acorns grow mighty oaks. I was ready to sow my seeds of intention and nurture it with faith, determination and dedication to achieve my goal.

My doctor and I set a realistic objective to bring down my blood glucose sugar levels. At the time of starting the program, my stats were Fasting - 200+, PP - 250+ and H1bAc at 10.3. We now aimed to bring it down to Fasting below 100, PP around 140 and H1bAc below 7 within the next three months. Considering my alarming blood sugar levels, I was advised medication for 15 to 30 days, maximum. Since the medical prescription had an upper time limit, I relented and agreed to follow through.

As far as I was concerned, I believe my determination to abstain from medication right from 2012 to 2019 led me to discover an alternate method of healing. So, a firm intention put out to the universe is paramount. And when you see a window of opportunity, take the leap of faith. Once you've chosen your path, stick to it with determination. Dedicate time, effort and energy for a routine that will work towards reaching your goals. If healing is holistic, recovery is significant.

Would this work? Time would tell.

Chapter 2 : SETTING THE REVERSAL GOALS

"Never quit. It is the easiest cop-out in the world. Set a goal and don't quit until you attain it. When you do attain it, set another goal, and don't quit until you reach it. Never quit".

Every journey must culminate at a destination. So also, every action must contribute to a constructive goal. I had decided to invest in my health and sowed the seeds of intent in the vast universe. Now came the part of setting realistic reversal targets.

I knew I had to action the following in the next three months.
- Stop medication within 15/30 days
- Bring down my fasting glucose levels to <100
- Ensure the PP was <140
- Move the HbA1c < 7

So, this was the 3 phase timeline for the 7-stage reversal goals.
- ✓ Stage 1 Reduce sugar levels, continue medication (1- 15 days max)
- ✓ Stage 2 Reduce sugar levels and medication. (15 - 30 days)
- ✓ Stage 3 When HbA1c > 6, stop medication
- ✓ Stage 4 Reduce HbA1c < 6
- ✓ Stage 5 Pass the GTT (Glucose Tolerant Test)
- ✓ Stage 6 Start reversal of complications

- ✓ Stage 7 Normal sugar levels for all meals with ultimate fitness levels.

To provide a solution, you need to understand the problem. Ergo, for the above to work, I first had to understand what didn't work and why? So, I decided to go back in time and analyse what piece did not fit in this 'sweet' puzzle.

As a diabetic patient, my diet before my FFD journey looked something like this.

6.30 am — One fruit before exercise

8.30 to 9.00 am — Tea and breakfast (Poha/Upma/Idli/Paratha)

11.00 am — Fruit

1.00 to 1.40 pm — Lunch (1-3 Chapati, Dal, Subji, Buttermilk and Salad)

4.00 pm — Tea with some snacks

6.30 pm — Fruit

8.0 to 9.00 pm — Dinner (similar to Lunch)

Bedtime — Milk

If you've understood anything about me till now, you'd know that I can be quite obstinate. And I was when it came to following this diet. Yet the perfect non-diabetic score continued to allude me despite my best intentions. Every well-meaning person advised me to eat less, but more frequently. Still, the six to eight meals a day simply weren't cutting it on the scoreboard.

That's the problem with anything half baked; it leaves you unsatiated and hungry.

Everything became crystal clear when the doctors at FFD explained that there were three primary reasons for high sugar levels in adults with Type II Diabetes.

1. Excess fat
2. Acidic and inflamed systems
3. Lack of micronutrients

What did it mean for my body?

Basic biology tells us that pancreas produce insulin which attaches to receptors present over the cell walls to facilitate the movement of sugar from the blood to the cell. However, the excess fat inside the muscle cells stops the sugar from being absorbed and causes insulin resistance. As a result, the sugar levels go up.

Our unhealthy diets make our body acidic, and the inflamed systems work against our predominantly alkaline mechanism.

Since we don't follow a balanced diet, micronutrients like Vitamin B12 and D3 also tend to be in the deficit.

In short, the core system is failing, and if you don't address it, everything else is temporary relief.

Understanding the functionality of the body made me realise how I wanted to address and overcome the issue. And it was no rocket science. I had to reduce excess fat, move my body parameters from acidic to alkaline and increase my intake of micronutrients. Simple, eh?

Not really.

Now came the battle plan.

It started with no entry for FAT in the system. Did you know that fat enters our system quietly through milk, curd, ghee, oil, (eggs, poultry and meat for non-vegetarians)? I always thought that 'fat-free' meant that it was, but clearly, I was wrong.

Every food item we consume has 1 to 2 teaspoons of oil, which calculates to almost 1 litre per person, per month. The ideal requirement is 300 ml per month.

We've all grown up on the benefits of drinking a glass of milk every day. Milk products are touted as healthy alternatives, too. However, confirmed tests on people who stopped the consumption of milk and dairy products showed a marked decline in their sugar levels.

My immediate task was to reduce my oil intake and stop all milk and dairy products.

Next in the strategy was to make my body more alkaline. Unhealthy, unchecked diets contribute to inflammation that deteriorates and damages the organs of the body. So, I made a list of all the acidic items and decided to bid them a fond farewell. Milk and dairy products were already number one on that list.

Cheese

Tea/Coffee

Wine

Vinegar, Salt (Excess)

Wheat (I love wheat but a man's gotta do what a man's gotta do.)

I don't consume any of the below items, but they are on the list. So, off they go.

Alcohol

Red meat

Poultry and Fish

It's not easy to put the brakes on an ongoing lifestyle, so ease your system into an improved routine. Start by reducing the intake of acidic foods. Switching to an alternative is another option, e.g. if you are addicted to cups of coffee or tea, switch to 1 – 2 cups of black coffee or tea with no sugar or milk. Green tea is a healthier choice.

Time	The Diabetic Diet Chart	The Freedom Diet chart
6 to 7 am	Tea/Coffee with milk, without sugar + biscuits	Stunning Nutrient Dense Green Smoothie, Black tea without milk or with coconut milk Green tea or Herbal tea or No tea
8 to 9 am	Poha/Upma /Idli/Omelette Paratha/Roti Sabji	No Grains breakfast. Sprouts (50% of breakfast) and/or bean-based e.g. Besan Dosa (chilla/tomato omelette) / Moong dal/Matki/Chawli dosa/Appe/Mix Whole daal Thalipeeth + green chutney
1 to 2 pm	Chapati + Pulses or Non veg + subji+ curd/ buttermilk	One Grain Lunch. Bhakri (Bajra/Jowar/Rajgira/Millets/Pearl Barley) / Chapati (30%) + Low /zero oil sabji (25%) + Dal (20%) + Salad (25%)
4 to 5 pm	Tea/Coffee with milk without sugar + biscuits + Snacks	Fruits/ Repeat Green Juice/ Healthy Snacks Soaked Almonds and Walnuts
7.30 to 8.30 pm	Same as Lunch	Dinner similar to lunch or Soup, Salad/Khichadi
		Sleep latest by 11 pm and
		Get Sleep for at least 7 hours

You probably already know this, but I'm going to say it anyway. Refined and processed food items are a strict no-no. So, say goodbye to maida, bread, cakes, biscuits, polished rice, etc.

Increasing micronutrients needed additional supplement solutions, administered under a doctor's prescription with careful monitoring. In layman's language, it's like boosting the system with anti-virus to protect and defend.

I've also added the FFD diet chart for those of you who'd like to follow it. Trust me when I tell you this; it's not that difficult. Once you sieve your lifestyle, you'll automatically filter the unhealthy options and make a better you with what remains.

Chapter 3 : BEING MINDFUL OF THE 3 PRONG PROCESS

"Do not dwell in the past, do not dream of the future, concentrate the mind on the present moment."

~ Buddha

The reversal goals had been set, and wheels of change set in motion. I took it one day at a time and made these lifestyle readjustments. Was it easy? Absolutely not! However, with each passing day, my rebellious body became accustomed to the new routine. I realised that to train the body you first have to train the mind in three areas; *food, exercise and monitoring.*

Food

I am a TEA totaller, and by that, I mean downing a minimum of 4 to 5 cups of tea with milk and little sugar. I thought that less or no sugar was good enough for my health not realising milk was the stealthy one. Once on the FFD diet, I switched to black tea and coffee (twice a day) continued my intake of Chinese/Herbal tea throughout the day.

I decided to stick with the three major meals of the day, breakfast, lunch and dinner. As per the chart, this was how my daily diet looked.

6 to 6.30 am Smoothie

8.30 to 9 am Breakfast

1 to 2 pm   Lunch

4 pm   Nuts (almonds and walnuts soaked in water for 2 hours)

6 pm   Smoothie

8 pm   Dinner

Now the SMOOTHIE is the catalyst in this story of change. As much as it didn't appeal to me in the beginning, as all new things are wont to do, today I swear by its benefits. Due to its massive green vegetables content, it adds the required fibre and oxygen to the body. 500 ml needs to be taken twice a day, in the am and the pm. It satiates those hunger pangs and keeps you on the path of wellness.

Smoothie recipe 500 ml

1 ½ cup chopped leaves with stems of any major green (Spinach, Kardai, Ambat Chutka, Amaranth green-red, Hemp/Ambadi etc.)

1 beetle leaf,

1 sprig of curry leaves

¼ cup of mint leaves

10 leaves of black tulsi

1/3 big apple or ¾ small apple or pear

1 tbs of lemon juice

A pinch of rock salt

1/4 tsp of cinnamon powder

¼ tsp of pepper powder

¼ tsp turmeric powder

Put everything in a mixer and churn for 3 minutes.

And voila, your tasty, healthy and refreshing smoothie is ready to drink.

Breakfast was 1 bowl of salad and 1 cup of dal based or grain-based item. So that would be 5 to 7 pcs of appam or 2 vadas or 1 chilla.

Lunch and dinner had a 25% formula. Essentially, you had to consume all your food items equally. So, that made it 25% each of Salad, Chapati/Rice, Dal and Sabji. If you ate an additional chapati, you had to consume the 2nd bowl of salad, dal and sabji to maintain the status quo.

Initially, the body seemed too hungry at times. And that's a given, considering the previous consumption patterns. However, slowly and steadily, the diet began to grow on the digestive system. Of course, you are allowed to eat chana, vatana, chana dal or makhana as a snack if you are hungry. That is the best part of this process. They never advocate starvation.

Exercise

The doctors advised me to adhere to a simple exercise routine for about 40 minutes to an hour.

a) 20 minutes of walk
b) Chair Suryanamaskar
   https://www.youtube.com/watch?v=9DGKdhJSc5Q&t=62s
c) Pranayams.

I also had to follow some anti-gravity and strength-building exercises.

1. Climbing stairs
   If your joints are fine, blood pressure is normal, and you have no heart problems, this can give you breakthrough results. 1 ½ hour after every meal start climbing up and down your stairs. Start by climbing one floor at a time (15-20 steps). Repeat and increase it steadily from 3-5 to 8-10 times. If you start panting, stop. Your PP reading will reduce by at least 20 points, and it also helps you lose weight.
2. Weight Training

It is recommended for 20 minutes, thrice a week, under the guidance of a professional trainer. It is an effective method to build muscle and burn fat.

Understanding the importance of the lymphatic movement

We all learned in school that arteries carry oxygenated blood from the heart to the tissues, while veins carry deoxygenated blood to the heart. Veins have valves and arteries have the blood pressure to guide their movement. Besides these two, lymphatic vessels carry lymph (fluid) directly to the heart. They don't have valves or pressure and depend solely on body movement. Hence, the non-movement of your body creates stagnation of the fluid and leads to inflammation. Do the following specific exercises to avoid this.

a. Dry rubbing
   Rub your entire body, one part at a time, with the help of a soft towel, gently.

b. Energy shake
   Shake different parts of the body in a step by step sequence; hands, legs,

spine, back, head, hair, tongue, wrists, arms and stomach.

c. Skipping/Trampoline

It is a recommended exercise as the upward workouts facilitate the lymph movement.

d. Swinging of hands and legs

Monitoring

Discipline will hold you in good stead and keep you on track. And that's why monitoring your progress is imperative. It helps you work out strategies in case you stumble or get slow. It also acts as a motivation to see a health scorecard that's on the upward swing.

You must monitor your blood sugar four times a day.

Fasting   Before meals

PP1   2 hours after breakfast

PP2   2 hours after Lunch

PP3   2 hours after dinner

Within the first week, my sugar levels started dropping, and I reduced my dosage from 4 tablets to 3. Another three days   and my medication was down to 2 tablets. Two weeks later, I was on ½ tablet of the least effective sugar medicine. As promised by the FFD team, within 15 days, I was on negligible medication. It felt like I had taken the best decision of my life.

I was now off maida, bread, milk, paneer, cheese, mayo, biscuits, canned juices, and tea/coffee with milk. I remember I had planned an 18-day family trip to Europe and had doubts about sticking to my diet. So, I apprehensively approached my doctor, and his advice was simple.

Try and eat as many vegetables as you can. Look for salads, wraps (although it has maida), fruits and vegan pizza. If you don't get a vegan pizza, then eat the one you find BUT DO NOT STARVE. The most important tip, ENJOY YOUR HOLIDAY and don't ruin it by running behind the diet. Remember, happiness is one of the biggest reasons that helps reduce sugar levels.

Believe me when I tell you it was one of my best vacations ever! We travelled across Denmark, Norway, Finland, Estonia and Sweeden, all exceptionally famous for   their dairy and confectionery. Yet, I didn't give in to temptation even a single day.

I followed my doctor's advice and enjoyed the salads, wraps on a few occasions, falafals, and many more items. I have an entire list of things to eat and avoid at the end of the book. However, the point I'm making is that I had the freedom to eat what I wanted. Yet, I had become so mindful of following the three-prong process of Food, Exercise and Monitoring, that it was an organic decision to abstain. Also, I must mention that I was on medication during this trip as a precaution.

On my return from my holiday, about 33 days after starting the FFD journey, the doctor asked me to stop my medication altogether. I can't describe that feeling to you. It was a vindication of my beliefs and my gift to my wellbeing.

The Diabetes App that I was following had the following parameters.

Blood test	Green	Orange	Red
Fasting	up to 100	100 to 120	120+

PP   up to 140   140 to 160   160+

So, green to orange was fine, but the moment I hit red, I had to readjust my diet to move back into the safe zone. My business required me to travel often, and it was another month of being on the FFD diet. Most of the time, I was in the safe zone, rarely crossing over to the red. No matter the stakes, I continued my diet and exercise. They had become a part of my lifestyle now.

Two months later, my stats looked something like this.

No medicine for sugar.

Hb1Ac   less than 8

Weight   from 86 to 82

So with level one of the transformation unlocked, it was time for phase 2.

Also, I must mention this.

Many have raised doubts about stopping milk as it may lead to a deficiency in Calcium, Protein, and Iron etc. When you look at the scientific data given below, you will understand as your body will experience that this path offers much better nutrition than your former consumption.

Greens are a rich source of protein and calcium. 51% of calories retrieved from spinach comes from protein, unlike the 10 to 15% that we assumed. Imagine the biggest mammals on land, elephants, giraffes, gorillas, pandas, hippos, rhinos, all of them survive and thrive on greens. We've been taught that milk, eggs and meat are better sources of protein, calcium, iron, etc., which isn't incorrect. However, greens, beans, pulses, nuts and seeds are equally excellent sources.

Protein content of food (grams per 100 cal protein)

Milk	10g	Cheese	16-40g
Spinach	26 g	Broccoli	13g
Lentils	7.8g	Black beans	6.7 g
Kidney beans	6.4g	Peas	6.4 g
Pumpkin seeds	5.2g	Amaranth (Rajgira)	3.8g
Pista	3.7g	Flax seeds	4.0g
Almonds	3.7g	Peanuts	4.3 g

Calcium content of foods (per 100-gram portion)

Human Milk	33 mg	Cow's milk	120mg
Spinach (Raw)	93 mg	Lettuce (dark green)	68 mg
Mustard Green (raw)	183 mg	Parsley	203 mg
Bhindi (Okra)	98 mg	Beans	135 mg
Chickpeas	150mg		
Almonds	234 mg	Amaranth	267 mg
Pista	131 mg	Raisins	62mg
Figs (dried)	126 mg	Sesame seeds	1160 mg
Sunflower seeds	120 gm	Orange	90mg

Iron-rich food

Add Beetroot, Broccoli, Dates, Raisins, Carrots, Sunflower seeds, Green Peas, Soya beans, Spinach, Almonds, Fenugreek, Figs, Tomatoes, Lentils, Chick Peas and Muesli to your diet to fight iron deficiency.

For Vitamin B12

Consume fermented items like Idli, Dosa, Dhokla, Yogurt (from plant milk), and Probiotic Drinks (Kanji) regularly to avoid B12 deficiency.

Remember to train the body and mind in the three-prong process of *food, exercise and monitoring.* Nothing works in isolation. Newton's law states that every action has an equal and opposite reaction. Ergo, with every progress you make, your sugar levels are receding. Just don't give up on yourself.

Chapter 4 : MAKING ROOM FOR THE NEW

"There are far, far better things ahead than any we leave behind."

The wheels of change were in motion, and they were slowly picking up momentum. The difference was visible, and I liked the change. I was following these three rules to the tee.

1. Eating three meals a day.
    a. Breakfast was a salad and sprout/dal based item or a grain-based item. Remember NO mixing of 2 grains ever. (Mixing of 2 or more grains tend to spike the sugar levels). So, you can't have Rice and Wheat /Jowar/Bajri in any one meal.
    b. Lunch and Dinner with the 25% formula. One bowl each of Salad, Dal and Sabji with one Chapatti or one bowl of rice (unrefined).
2. Skipping dairy products ALTOGETHER. Yes, I had become a Vegan.
3. Exercising for 1 hour every day comprising of walking, Surya Namaskars and Pranayams.

On achieving this stage, my confidence levels soared. I was raring to go and break some new milestones, and I knew what the next goal would be. I wanted to break the jinx of

78 kgs or less. I had never been below 78 kgs since my marriage in 1989, and all my attempts to achieve that magical weight had been nought. However, this time I had a feeling this could be it. The Law of Attraction works when you work at it, and this time I felt ready. It was time to make room for a new and improved me.

Let Phase 2 begin.

Now is where we accelerate the reversal process. I got a heads-up that it was going to get a bit bumpy. Well, I didn't quite understand that because there were just two crucial steps to follow.

1. Juice Feasting
2. Long Fasting

Well, I loved the first bit already! What wasn't to love? There were fruits, and there were juices, right?

Wrong.

Juice Feasting had nothing to do with fruits, except for the one in the smoothie. To the uninitiated, Juice Feasting or JF as we call it, is skipping all your meals (solid food) and spending your day only on different juices made out of multiple vegetables. Yes, you heard that right. Vegetables.

Well, at first glance I thought this was going to be a deal-breaker because how do you satiate yourself? I was pretty convinced I'd need to eat something by late evening. Surprisingly, I endured. Here's why and how.

A typical Juice Feasting day's routine is as under

�����������������

6 - 6.30 am   Smoothie
8.00 am   RED Juice
10.00 am   GREEN Juice 1
1.00 pm   GREEN Juice 2
3 - 3.30 pm   TANGY juice
6.00 pm   Smoothie
8.0 pm   White Juice

As you can see, the day is divided into multiple times that you can have a juice, and trust me, you survive. I was so full the first time that I skipped the white juice altogether.

Juice Feasting is one of the most potent and practical ways to shift the leptin resistance that is the root cause of obesity and Diabetes. Here is what it does.

- Detoxifies your body
- Packs your body with lots of nutrients
- These nutrients repair, cleanse and heal your body
- The digestive system gets some rest
- Helps to reset our physiology

In short, Juice Feasting Cleanses, Rebuilds, Rehydrates and Alkalises the body. Consume 4-5 litres of fresh, green, low glycaemic, preferably organic living juices in a day. Drink 2-3 glasses at 1.5 -2 hours intervals as one becomes hungry. The correct method is to eat these juices, i.e. roll every morsel in the mouth and chew before gulping it down.

Avoid strenuous exercise on Juice Feasting Day. You may do light exercise or rest on the day. Please choose a day when you do not have too much work and can get a lot of rest. Do bear in mind that you may visit the washroom multiple times.
You can try half-day of juice feasting and eat regular meals in the evening. You can even alternate between juices with fibre and non-fibre, as per your suitability. Remember, we are feasting and not fasting. So, adopt whatever suits your system best.

You can also have a cup of herbal tea or soup. If you are still starving, eat a handful of sprouts or soaked nuts. You might experience light headaches, unexplained feelings or mild diarrhoea. Don't worry, all these reactions are an essential part of the detoxification process, and will disappear soon. Keep checking your sugar levels at every 3-4 hours intervals.

Here are the crucial Dos and Don'ts of Juice Feasting.

- DON'T USE THE JUICER MIXER, but instead, DO USE A COLD PRESS JUICER.
- DON'T add water to the juices at all
- DO use all vegetables with the peel or edible stem, for juicing.
- DO clean and wash the vegetables thoroughly in turmeric and salt water before use.
- DO check the output while extracting juices and add vegetables as needed. DON'T put all the veggies in one go.

Now for the Juice Recipes.

RED JUICE: To be taken   between 8.00 am to 9.00 am

- 800 gm Tomato/ Tamatar
- 250 gm Carrots/ Gajar
- 1 red capsicum/ Laal Simla Mirch/ Laal Simla Mirchi
- 1 yellow capsicum/ Peeli Simla Mirch/ Pivli Simla Mirchi
- 1 pc. Ginger/ Adrak/ Ala
- Salt & Pepper as per your taste/ Namak, Kali Mirch, swaad anusar / Meeth, Kali Miri chavinusar

GREEN JUICE 1: To be taken between 11.00 am and 12.00 pm.

- 500 gm Ash Gourd/ Kohala/ Petha
- ½ apple/ Seb/ Safarchand
- 4 big green capsicums/ Badi Hari Simla Mirch/ Motthi Hirvi Simla Mirchi
- 1 ridge gourd/ Tori/ Dodka
- ½ lemon juice/ Nimbu ka ras/ Limbacha ras
- 1 pc. Ginger/ Adrak/ Ala

- Salt & Pepper as per your taste/ Namak, Kali Mirch, swaad anusar / Meeth, Kali Miri chavinusar

GREEN JUICE 2: To be taken between 1.30 pm and 2.30 pm.

- 700 gm Bottle gourd/ Lauki/ Dudhi
- 2 cups Chakavat/Aambatchuka/ Bathua/ Cholai or any edible leafy green
- 1 cup Coriander/ Hara dhania/ Kothimbir
- Lemon Juice/ Nimbu ka ras/ Limbacha ras
- 1 pc. Ginger/ Adrak/ Ala
- Salt & Pepper as per your taste/ Namak, Kali Mirch, swaad anusar / Meeth, Kali Miri chavinusar

TANGY JUICE: Can be taken as an alternative to Green Juice 2 - between 3.30 pm and 4.30 pm.

- 600 gm Bottle gourd/ Lauki/ dudhi
- 100 gm Cabbage/ Patta Gobhi/ Paan Kobi
- 4 Cucumber/ Khira/ Kakdi
- Lemon Juice/ Nimbu Ka Ras/ Limbacha Ras

- 1 pc. Ginger/ Adrak/ Ala
- Salt & Pepper as per your taste/ Namak, Kali Mirch, swaad anusar / Meeth, Kali Miri chavinusar

WHITE JUICE: Take between 7 pm to 8 pm

- 500 gm Bottle Gourd/ Dudhi/ Lauki
- 500 gm Cucumber/ Khira/ Kakdi
- Lemon Juice/ Nimbu Ka Ras/ Limbacha Ras
- 1 pc. Ginger/ Adrak/ Ala
- Salt & Pepper as per your taste/ Namak, Kali Mirch, swaad anusar / Meeth, Kali Miri chavinusar

As much as I thought I would be unable to do the Juice Feasting, I was pleasantly surprised. I'm now accustomed to the process as it is a great energy booster. I find my whole body becomes light, the system feels clean, and my skin starts glowing. The weight loss is a given.

The second part of this phase was prolonged fasting.

As a foodie, it simply wasn't my forte. However, I was doing things I never thought I would in my lifetime. I was invested, and the evident results drew me in further. I did the fasting across a 4-week interval.

1st Week - JF-3-2-3-2-3-2

That's no cryptic text. It merely means that the next day of Juice Feasting, I must have three regular meals consisting of Breakfast, Lunch and Dinner. The following day, I must have any two meals and drop either one from the trio as per my convenience. The pattern continues through the remainder of the week.

2nd Week - JF-2-2-2-2-2-2

Throughout the week, I am to have any two meals in the day. This week prepares the body to fast.

3rd Week - JF-2-1-2-1-2-1

In the third week, it came down to one meal a day for three our six days in a week. I was now fasting for 16 to 24 hours a day, minimum. It was indeed an eye-opener because I never thought I had it in me to fast so effortlessly. I was free from medication and wanted to go for a Jalebi test, but I digress. Let's get to week 4.

4th Week - JF-1-1-1-1-1-1.

I was now down to one meal a day! Effectively, I was fasting for 24 hours a day for the whole week. Smoothies and soaked nuts with 2 cups of herbal/black tea without sugar were my only other indulgence.

And what do you know, I broke the jinx of harbouring around 78 Kgs, finally!

No one could believe it, including me. My family thought I'd give in. I never thought I could do it in the first place though I was up for the challenge. The FFD diet prepares you one day at a time, giving your body, mind and soul time to adjust to a paradigm shift that changes everything.

5th week - JF -0-0-0-0-0-0- LONG FAST.

Now came the litmus test of the long fast. It was the most crucial phase, and I decided to take it one day at a time. The first 24 hours would tell if I had it in me make it to the finish line.

The 1st day was fine, and I could manage with little hunger and negligible food craving. Sipping on hot water helped me suppress my food cravings.

The 2nd day was tough, and by evening it looked as though I'd give up. Somehow, I gave myself a pep talk and carried on. I had been without solid food for 48 hours. My sugar levels were between 80 and 85 whilst fasting, and PP was 110-125.

On the 3rd day, my blood sugar fasting plummeted to 65. The doctor suggested eating two dates, and it then rose to 83. By the pm, the PP levels dropped to 69. Once again, I was asked to eat two dates immediately and test my sugar levels after 15 minutes. It was back to 85+. The doctor confirmed that my body was responding to fasting, which is essential in reversing the sugar levels.

4th day was under control.

I would have continued had it not been for an important family function. I broke my fast after 108 hours but learned that the human body could achieve wondrous things when challenged and pushed under the guidance of a trained eye.

At the end of Phase 2, my blood glucose levels were under control without medicine. It had been 2 ½ months, and at 78 Kgs, I was lighter by 8 kgs, too.

Sugar levels   Fasting 90 to 95   PP 115 to 135

I had done it!

When something is meant to come your way, the universe will conspire to make it happen. Just remember to make room for the change. I owe my gratitude to the universe, the FFD team, my family and friends who have been the supporting cast in my magnum opus.

Let the good times roll in.

Chapter 5 : GETTING RID OF THE OLD

"A man will be imprisoned in a room with a door that's unlocked and opens inwards; as long as it does not occur to him to pull rather than push".

I felt like a brand-new man with Phase 1 and 2 accomplished. 8 out of 10 times my sugar was within the regular readings. At times, it would fluctuate due to a change in my food intake. However, it would come back within parameters, and all this without medication. I was a happy man with my achievements.

Time to unlock Phase 3, the transformation of the mind.

Did you know that one of the significant reasons for Diabetes is mental stress? I recommend listening and reciting the following prayers every day in the morning and evening for calm and peace.

(Prayer - NEEDS TO BE ADDED) * Its an audio file .. will provide link*

The transformation of the mind begins with a change in attitude. You have to accept who you are, acknowledge what you want to let go, appreciate where this journey might lead you and affirm why you need to do this, over and over again.

Sow the seeds of these attributes, and watch your life take a turn for the better.

1. Have Gratitude.
2. Always Forgive
3. Learn to Forget
4. Nissprund Devo Bhava
5. Love yourself
6. Love the universe
7. Love what you do or do what you love

1. Have Gratitude.

Simple words like *'Thank you'*, *'I appreciate it'*, *'I am grateful'* are excellent relationship builders. One must cultivate being thankful for all that you have and are for our well being. Remember to love yourself and keep room for consideration for others. Be kind. It costs nothing and is a great personality enhancer.

Take a minute to recall every person that has contributed to your journey. Pen a thank you note to all of them. Acknowledge that you are the sum of many experiences made of people, places and things. Don't forget to say thank you to yourself. There is just one of your kind. Make that note special.

You will find at least 50 people you owe your gratitude to with this exercise. Parents, family, siblings, children, friends, colleagues, teachers, neighbours, childhood crushes, city, country, and the universe must have brought you some joy. Connect with them and let them know they matter, and that you are grateful for their presence in your life.

Make it a ritual to thank at least five people every day and witness the glow of happiness on their faces or in their voices.

2. Always Forgive.
   Anger, hurt, hey and resentment are unnecessary baggage we carry that make our journey exhausting. They add to your mental stress and physical trauma. In the wise words of Elsa, 'Let it go'.

Whatever is bothering you is in the past, done and dusted. Why waste the present and the future on it? You can't change it, but you can change your reaction to it. Being able to forgive is the mark of strength and magnanimity. It shows that you are willing to go past human behaviour and be the bigger person.

Do this for yourself. And for the other person because nothing brings more peace than a forgiving heart.

3. Learn to Forget

    If you forgive, but don't forget you are not moving forward. Learning to forget is a crucial step to forgiving. Harbouring a need for revenge slows down the healing process. We focus our energy in the wrong direction for the wrong reasons, and we tend to move away from our goals. In our mission to teach the other person a lesson, we might lose focus from what truly matters to us. And this time will never come back.

We need to make room for newer experiences, and holding on to the past makes it difficult. Of course, our lives will have their fair share of disappointments, broken hearts and shut doors. However, take it in your stride, keep the lesson and let go of everything else. When you forgive and forget, you will feel begin to feel lighter, like the lifting of a heavy load. Cherish this feeling because nothing matters more than your mental, physical and emotional well-being.

4. Nissprund Devo Bhava (Getting detached)

It stems from the act to forgive and forget and urges one on the path of acceptance. Only in the wisdom of acceptance do you understand that you are not responsible for whatever happens in the world. It's your calling to do your part and not worry about the consequences. Karma traces the path of every action.

In this enlightened sense of detachment, accept all that comes on your path with open arms and let it go with a smile. Do not try to hold on to anything because it is futile. What rises must fall and what comes must go. It might sound complicated, but it is easy once you understand that you are a speck in the universe of things. Be in the now and be free of *moha* and *maya.* You will realise that things cease to affect you, and that is the path of wholesomeness.

5. Love yourself.

    I can't stress this enough. How can you fill others with happiness and joy if you are empty? You must nurture yourself to be able to give of your heart, freely. When was the last time you did something that you liked? How many times do you appreciate you? How many times do you judge yourself?

    Let's do a little exercise to make this clearer. Be as honest as you can.

Things you like about yourself	Things you don't like about yourself

Which list is longer? If it's the one on the left, keep doing whatever it is that you are doing. However, if it's the one to your right, then cut yourself some slack. Own your life, your path, your good, your not so good, and all that goes with it. You are the only one of your kind, and you are perfect just the way you are.

6. Love the universe.

See all the abundance surrounding you. Be grateful for the generations that came before you, be hopeful for the ones that will come after you.

Make your life count, and count all the priceless moments you've had in your life. The cosmos responds to your vibe, so choose a happy song.

Challenges are a part of the process. Be brave to answer the call, and the universe will conspire. Be love and give love.

7. Love what you do or do what you love.
    You are lucky if you do what you love. And you are luckier if you love what you do. It is my eternal Guru Mantra in life. Enjoy where you are to the fullest, and you won't feel the stress. If you lament and mourn for what could have been, you'll be miserable.

    Remember, you always have a choice. Find a win-win option. It won't be easy, then again all worthwhile things never are. It's your life; make it grand.

These seven steps have unveiled a sense of newness in my life. I realised that the outside influences the inside and vice versa. To be genuinely free of disease, you need a sacred union between the body, mind and soul. The mind is the most difficult to control, and yet that is where healing is the strongest. Learn to master the reaction, and the action will bear fruit in its due course.

Chapter 6 : ESTABLISHING A NEW SUGAR-FREE ROUTINE

"The first step to living the life you want is leaving the life you don't want".

Karen Salmansohn

Once you've decided to mend your old ways, you will need help. Always ask for it. Nothing happens in isolation, so look for your tribe and hold on to them. I know I did.

In my journey to be medication-free, I had to take adequate measures. For starters, I had to know what my diabetic parameters were to work on reducing them. These are the tests that you need to do. Do consult your medical practitioner for a more personalised recommendation.

LIST OF IMPORTANT TESTS:

1. Blood Sugar-Fasting & PP

2. HbA1C

3. Lipid profile

4. Hemogram

5. Vitamin B12

6. Vitamin D3

7. Liver Function Tests

8. Kidney Function Tests with Glomerular Filtration Rate (eGFR)

9. Thyroid Function Tests

10.Urine Routine and Urine microalbumin

11. Iron Study

12. High Sensitive C-Reactive Protein (hsCRP)

13. Fasting Insulin

In the case of Type 1 Diabetics, get your C peptide (Fasting and PP) done as well.

I did the above tests at 3-month intervals to rule out other complications. Fortunately, barring blood pressure, everything was under control. However, issues like Thyroid, PCOD, Fibroids, Weight Gain and Weight loss accompany Diabetic profiles.

I was now at Phase 4, where my HbA1c was < 6 sans medication. I decided to maintain the same for another three months for my body to adjust to these levels before I went for stage 5 of the GTT (Glucose Tolerance Test).

During these three months, I decided to become fitter under the advice of Dr Malhar.

I had lost 16 kgs of fat with diet and exercise, but he now advised me to gain muscle. He prescribed the following exercise routine.

1. 25 Suryanamaskars
2. 7 Resistance band exercises with 3 sets of repetition
3. Core exercise to reduce the belly fat
4. Weights to increase muscle

My mentor Ms Vasudha Chavan motivated me further. She began running at the age of 60 and in 3 years she went on to run 42 half marathons. It was difficult to believe that at one point in time, she was on strong medication, including insulin. A superhero, indeed. Her real-life transformation egged me into thinking that if she could do it, I could too.

I followed the thumb rule by Dr Malhar, *'Diet to reduce weight and exercise to tone your body'*.

My exercise routine looked something like the pictures that follow. On alternate days I did the 25 Suryanamaskars.

I had an easy diet as I was now 73 kgs with a BMI of 24. My next goal was to weigh 68 Kgs with the HbAc1 < 6.

Getting to where I was might have seemed impossible a few months ago. Yet, a paradigm shift in the thinking was all that   it took for change to happen. Bring in the new when the old ceases to be of value. My new sugar-free routine has made my life sweeter, pun intended.

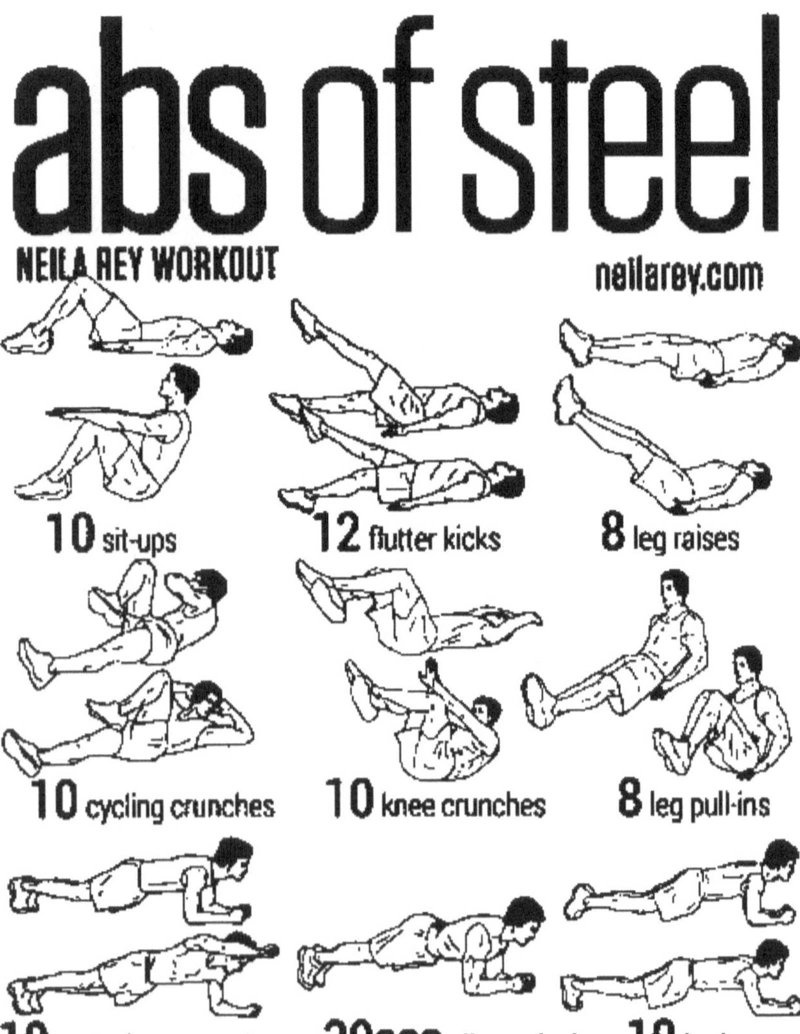
abs of steel
NEILA REY WORKOUT
neilarey.com
10 sit-ups
12 flutter kicks
8 leg raises
10 cycling crunches
10 knee crunches
8 leg pull-ins
10 e/plank arm reaches
30sec elbow plank
10 body saw

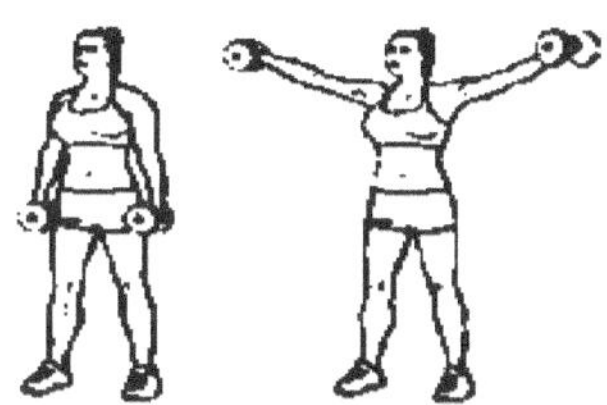

Lateral / Side Shoulder
Dumbbell Raises / Power
2 sets / 12 reps

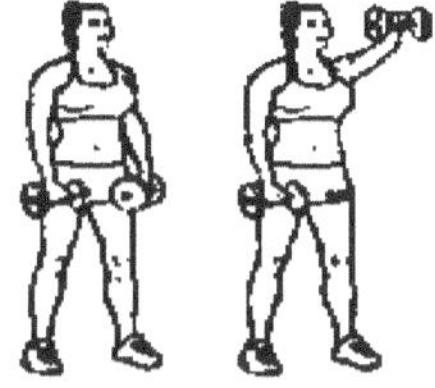

Forward / Front Shoulder
Dumbbell Raises
2 sets / 12 reps

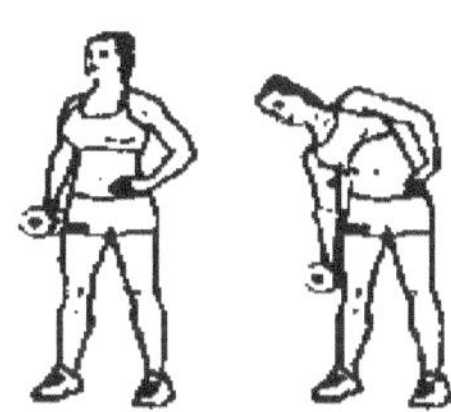
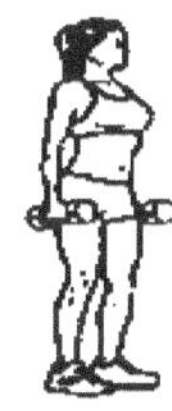

Standing Dumbbell /
Kettlebell Side Bends
2 sets / 12 reps

Standing Dumbbell Bicep
Curls
2 sets / 12 reps

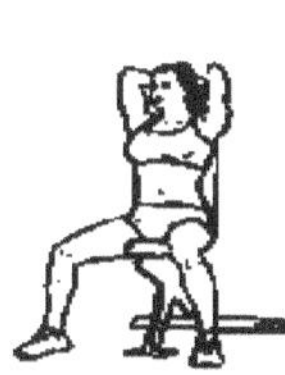
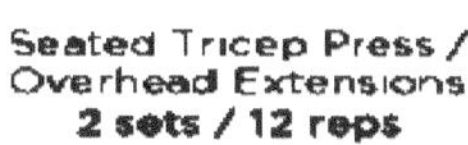
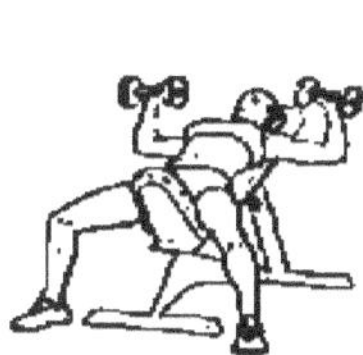
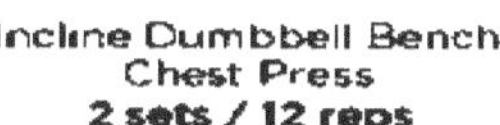

Seated Tricep Press /
Overhead Extensions
2 sets / 12 reps

Incline Dumbbell Bench
Chest Press
2 sets / 12 reps

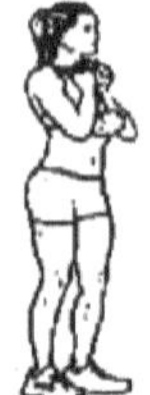
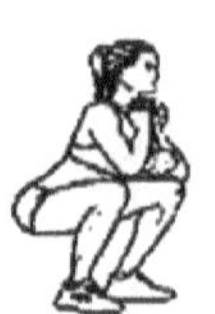

Goblet Squat
3 sets / 15 reps

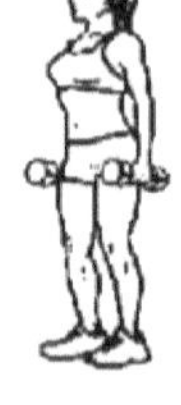

Dumbbell Side Lunge /
Lateral Lunge
3 sets / 10 reps

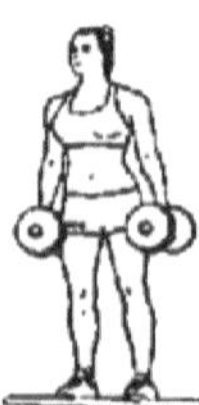
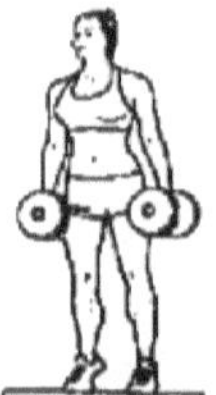

Standing Dumbbell Calf
Raise
3 sets / 20 reps

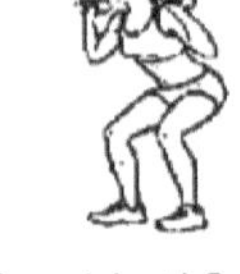

Dumbbell Squat Thrusters /
Squat to Overhead Press
3 sets / 20 reps

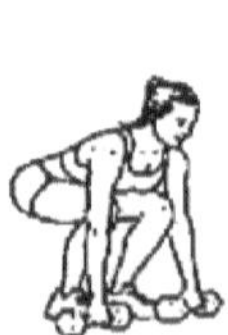

Dumbbell Deadlift
3 sets / 10 reps

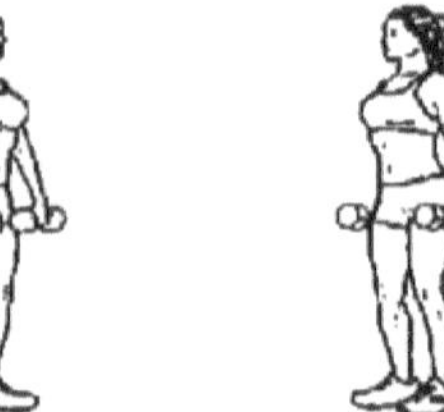
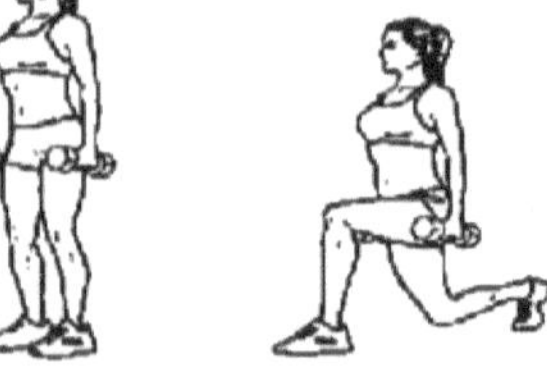

Dumbbell Lunges
3 sets / 10 reps

Epilogue : REDISCOVERING THE REAL SWEETNESS OF LIFE

"Find the sweetness in your own heart; then you may find the sweetness in every heart".

I am at the last leg of my Sugar-Free Journey in this book. My (Hb1Ac) reading for the past 3 months has been around 6, and I am off medicine since the past year. I have another blood test before the Glucose Tolerance Test. However, my sustained efforts in managing my diet now allow me the occasional sweets and savouries in a limited quantity. I am stringent about exercising for 4-5 times a week, and my routine is now more of a lifestyle.

1. 6.00 - 7.00 am   200 ml smoothie with half fruit
2. 7.00 - 8.30 am   Exercise Superbrain yoga (10 situps x 3 times) Squats (15 x 3)

Yoga comprising of some asanas, anulom vilom, kapalbhati

and savasana Alternate days 36/48 surya namaskars

or Abs of steel Once a week,

long walk /climb stairs (13 stories)/jogging to break the routine.

3. 9.00 am   Breakfast Dal based food with Salad and sprou (Please check with your dietician for your nutrition)
4. 10.30 - 11 am   Black tea without sugar
5. 1.00 to 1.30   Lunch. 25% formula of salad, roti, dal and sabji
6. 4.00 pm   Black coffee without sugar
7. 6.00 - 7.00 pm   Light snack of Chana/Vatana/Makhana or smoothie
8. 8.00 - 9.00 pm   Dinner same as Lunch

I take weekly readings to monitor my parameters. Due to my vegan diet and my exercise routine, I was advised to take a protein supplement. I take 30 gms of Unived pea protein powder with water after my daily exercise.

Here is a quick recap if you are planning on starting your sugar-free journey today. Please bear in mind, follow the advice under the guidance of qualified doctors.

1. Sow the intention with a positive mind to see yourself free from medicine as soon as possible.
2. Once you've made up your mind, follow it up with the right actions. Consult the right doctors and follow the appropriate therapy with proven results.
3. Follow the advice with dedication and determination.
4. Set realistic goals, fix your timelines and adjust your schedule.
5. Follow the diet.
6. Do the exercises.
7. Give your body, mind and soul the permission to release all negativity. Let it all go and feel a soul cleanse.
8. Monitor your goals periodically and make adjustments to meet short term goals via a change in diet or exercise.

Know that help is available, and the universe is conspiring. Trust yourself and take that leap of faith. And you will find that doors unlock and windows open, as the fresh air and light make their way into your life.

Believe, and it's yours.

In Gratitude

I would like to thank the following people who made this journey possible, with every little milestone. I am indeed lucky to call them my tribe.

The biggest thank you to the Almighty for this journey and for blessing me with everything that I have today.

I am indebted to my wife, Bina Shah, who is the better half in this relationship and my rock of Gibraltar. If it weren't for her steadfast belief in me, I would have given up a long time ago. Now, she enjoys the smoothies and occasional vegan desserts.

My sons, Krish and Parth, have supported and encouraged me throughout my journey, and I am proud to know they have my back.

My angel in disguise and the brain behind Freedom From Diabetes, Dr Pramod Tripathi is a fantastic personality. He gives every patient his time and expertise with a smile on his face. Dr Pramod understands it is not easy, and every patient is on a personal journey. Hence, he leads you gently into the system, and the whole experience becomes one of self-discovery.

All the qualified mentors and doctors at the Freedom From Diabetes organisation, ever ready to help, and are just a phone call away.

Dr Malhar, the triathlon man, you motivated me into correctly toning my body.

My family doctor, Dr Hemang Nanavati, you believed in me, and that made this a possibility.

My batch colleagues, it is your camaraderie that enabled me to work along with you on this life-changing experience.

Mr Suresh Manshiramani for your guidance and encouragement to write this book without which I wouldn't have taken the plunge.

Dear Readers, thank you for choosing to learn more about my experience. I do hope I have been able to shift some thinking to help you choose a better lifestyle. I'd be happy to answer any queries or questions that you might have. Do write to me on hitech456@gmail.com

Also, if you could leave your feedback/review on your purchase site, I'd be grateful.

Thank you, and stay healthy, always.

Parag Shah

Appendix I

<u>Always Remember</u>

- The most crucial asset that you have in this life is your BODY.
- You have ONLY ONE BODY for your entire life.
- Your body is IRREPLACEABLE and therefore
- The better the body is, the HAPPIER are you and your inner circle.
- When in doubt remember that if you don't look after your body, it won't hold you in good stead as the years pass by.

Appendix II

<u>Travel diet plans - Planning for a trip/relatives/occasions</u>

Most plans are known well in advance. Hence you can plan to carry with you all/ many of the following essentials.

- Optional Small Hand Blender and small rice cooker
- Plastic containers to carry cooked millets
- Millets, Sprouts (sprouted and otherwise) in a wet cloth in a Ziploc bag
- Leafy vegetables wrapped in a wet cloth in a Ziploc bag
- Turmeric powder, cinnamon powder, pepper powder, rock salt, sesame seeds, Smoothie mix masala and dried leafy veg powders
- Raw cucumber, tomatoes, capsicum and carrots
- Roasted chana dal, moong dal
- Sunflower seeds, Cucumber seeds, other assorted seeds

- Dry chutneys
- Walnuts and almonds in small containers (soaked the previous night)
- Makhna
- Chana and moong jor
- Thalipeeth powder
- Besan/moong dal dough for 1 day
- Chorafali Khakra
- THERA BAND for workouts

Staying in a HOTEL in India

- Find out the hotel telephone numbers in advance and discuss your diet requirement for the day of arrival. Even otherwise, as soon as you check-in, connect with the kitchen and let them know about your dietary needs. Give them adequate time to prepare your food.
- Most chefs oblige and cook as per your dietary requirements
- Check out the ingredients of each item and restrict the use of oil in cooking

- Minimise the oil as far as possible. Check for the use of cold-pressed oils.
- You can carry your own cooked millets/oats/barley with you
- You can have chutneys, salad, clear soups –Lemon coriander, Lung Fung Veg soup, tomato shorba etc (No paneer)
- Plain dal, Boiled veg, Sprout salad, Stir-fried veggies, Boiled Matki (part of Misal –without the oil and PAV)
- Methi dal or Dal Palak without oil
- Medu Wada (strain the oil by using paper napkins or dipping in hot water) with lots of veggies in sambhar and coconut chutney
- Roasted Papad or Roasted Masala Papad
- Boiled Kabuli chana / Rajma (add to salads)
- Boiled peanuts in a minimum quantity are OK, as they are acidic
- Avoid refined rice and maida preparations
- Avoid grains
- Pesarattu (made of Moong dal) OR Adaiin South India (check that there is no rice in the same)

- Check ingredients of Tomato Omelette as it sometimes contains rice flour
- Have missi roti, tawa wheat roti or tandoori roti
- In Maharashtra, Gujarat, Rajasthan we get jowar, bajra rotis also. Pithale-bhakri (besan ki sabzi), daal–baati (no ghee) with lots of green salad, pickle and roasted daal papad.
- In South India, we get multiple millets' items.
- In many cities, there are VEGAN Restaurants.
- Some hotels have barley dishes and rotis as well as brown rice items
- Avoid any rich gravies having cream, curds, paneer and khoya or made in ghee or butter
- Avoid vegetables having fruits in them. Order simple vegetables like bhindi, matar, cauliflower, cabbage, Capsicum, baingan
- Avoid potato at all costs.
- Mushroom-Matar, shaslik (tandoori mushroom), Barbecued vegetable, Vegetable stew, Oats porridge (lunch/dinner) Veg clear soups (no sweet corn). Many hotels offer

sprouts, soaked lobhiya (chavli)matki missal on request

- Misal without poha, potato and bun-bread in a bowl with lots of onion, tomato, coriander, lemon, little or no farsan
- Moong dal pakodas/wada, Chana daal wada, vegetable pakoda
- No potato/cheese /paneer/Tandoori mushroom.
- Soak out the oil in paper napkins.
- Chaat items without puris, puffed rice and potato patties
- INTERMITTENT FASTING is a good option-breakfast and dinner

If you do not get food according to your requirements, BE READY TO COMPROMISE WITH AVAILABLE FOOD. DO NOT FEEL GUILTY, ESPECIALLY AS YOU HAVE MADE YOUR BEST EFFORTS. Do not get perturbed with fluctuating sugar levels. They will stabilise over a few days.

<u>Visiting Relatives or friends in India</u>

- Do not feel shy to explain your situation thoroughly. Inform them in advance of your dietary requirements. They are family and friends, after all. They will understand, sooner or later.
- Also hearing about your improvements in health will enthuse them to try the new food out and may help in their health problems as well.
- Try and AVOID too many exceptions.
- Carry snacks, Dal khakra/chorafali (without wheat), cooked millets etc., with you
- They can make smoothies for you if you carry the ingredients.

<u>Going to Weddings/ Conferences & Seminars and other occasions</u>

- Carry your cooked grains if possible
- You will get green salad, chutney and dal
- Dal may have oil, so you may have to adjust
- If you cannot carry your cooked grains, eating wheat roti is better than taking naan made of maida

- Take clear soups and check that for no cream or milk ingredients
- You could carry your lunch and afternoon smoothie with you
- Carry assorted seeds as well as some snacks for those cravings

For Holiday Travel Abroad

- Airline food is mostly UNHEALTHY so best to carry your food in flight
- Google search what leafy veggies are available in the country of travel
- Talk to your travel agent and check what the hotels can and cannot provide
- Talk to Hotel chefs where you are going to stay well in advance and check what adjustments they can do for you.
- Most hotel chefs will oblige you by making a smoothie with leafy veggies and any local fruit. Mostly, apple and pears are available
- Carry suitable and sufficient snacks if you are going to be on the road for most of the day
- Most Hotels have a reasonably large BUFFET breakfast including salads, fruits, steamed vegetables and some healthy soups too

- If possible, follow INTERMITTENT FASTING having only healthy breakfast and dinner
- If you plan and discuss with the chef, your dinner can also be VERY HEALTHY
- In the worst-case scenario, make adjustments but only to the extent necessary
- Ensure that you avoid Milk and Milk products. (Check ingredients in each dish carefully)

Going to stay with relatives abroad

- You can take a sprout maker to make moong and matki sprouts for breakfast.
- You can carry ATTA of Jowar, Bajri and Khapli Gehu from INDIA.
- You cannot carry millets or other grains, so look for substitutes. You will always get grains like Quinoa, Buckwheat, Steelcut oats, Barley etc.
- Google search and find out what leafy veggies are available to make your SMOOTHIE. Almost any green leafy veg will do EXCEPT SPINACH which is to be had ONLY ONCE A WEEK.

- Try to use expeller pressed /cold-pressed oils rather than processed or refined oils.
- Staying with relatives is a lot easier than when holidaying abroad.
- Plan as far as possible to minimise inconvenience to you, your family and most importantly your body.